Yoga and Resistance Bands

Dr. Victoria Coven

ISBN:978-1500539238

DEDICATION

This book is dedicated to all my students young and old. Their commitment to their yoga and strength training practice has fundamentally influenced their mental and physical health and touched those around them through its positivity.

CONTENTS

Acknowledgments

ACKNOWLEDGMENTS

I should like to acknowledge the teachers at the Esther Myers studio in Toronto. They showed me an interpretation of yoga that I believe has its essence in human being's relationship with the earth that we all stand upon. In this simplicity there is a freedom to adapt movements to suit all ages and abilities.

CHAPTER 1

Introduction

The resistance band is an exciting way to challenge any student's basic yoga practice. Once reserved solely for rehabilitation settings the resistance band is now a staple piece of equipment in the sports and fitness industry. Using the band for yoga brings a multitude of benefits. Firstly the resistance band introduces strength training to classical yoga. When any muscle meets a new level of resistance it responds with increased force and added effort. This added effort promotes muscle growth. In this way a resistance band adds challenge to traditional yoga postures (asanas). As we age there is a decline in muscle mass and strength which may effect ones quality of life. However using resistance bands can delay and even reverse this deterioration. Resistance bands can also slow or halt the normal loss of bone density that occurs with age and help prevent the resulting condition called osteoporosis. In normal free weight training you are limited to the amount of weight that you can lift at the weakest point in the exercise. For instance when you are doing a full squat you find the weak point occurs when you bend your knees at about 140 degrees and that you are getting stronger as you reach the top part of the movement. Resistance bands increase their resistance as they are stretched. This allows you to increase strength through a whole range of motion by loading the muscle at the end of the range of motion where it is strongest. The resistance bands may also be used for increasing the range of motion in flexibility poses. We can wrap the band around the feet, or hold our hands behind our back to increase flexibility in our whole body. The body will 'pull away' from the resistance offered by the band and will move in an increased range of motion, more so than if the traditional posture or asana was practiced with no band. This increased muscle usage releases increased endorphins into the bloodstream and gives us an increased sense of wellbeing and 'achievement' during exercise. Indeed, my first motivation for incorporating resistance bands into my yoga classes was for this sensation. I am an experienced yoga practitioner of many years and have taught extensively both in North America and the United Kingdom. I have always worked in fitness settings where yoga is just one exercise option for members. I found that students were foregoing the physical and mental health benefits that yoga offers because they simply didn't feel that they had worked their bodies hard enough during a yoga class. Using the bands releases the endorphins that the students needed to feel they achieved their fitness goals. Simultaneously they could experience the classical relaxation, meditative and flexibility promoting benefits of yoga, while developing strength within their bodies.

CHAPTER 2

The Three Principles of Yoga: The Ground, Breath and the Spine

I underwent yoga teacher training at the prestigious yoga studio Esther Myers in Toronto, Canada. This was the first studio established in this big city, which is of course now the home to a great number of such establishments each with their own styles, theories and doctrines. The philosophy offered at Esther Myers was organic, natural and simple. Esther Myer's teacher was Vanda Scarvelli and 3 ideas were to be borne in mind when carrying out each posture or asana. If these 3 principles were adhered to each student could then make the pose their own and adapt it to their own particular physical needs.

The Ground: Stability in each pose is established through a student feeling and understanding their relationship with the force of gravity. This means that there is no tension between this force and the body and therefore minimum effort is expended. To understand your relationship with the earth simply stand bare foot, and then sink your feet downward, experiencing the firm support of the ground. Try and grow 'roots'. Having a secure physical foundation will help you to feel more at ease emotionally. Notice how those under great emotional stress are unsteady on their feet. Anchor yourself during the poses and physical and emotional stability come forward to meet you. Experience this simple relationship with gravity in whatever part of your body happens to have contact with the ground for the pose that you are in. For example, in a sitting twist it is your sitting bones and in shoulderstand your shoulders. Once you can feel and appreciate this natural relationship, you can then move the rest of your body away from the force of gravity and create opening, lengthening and release. Every moment we are all in contact with the power of gravity that holds the earth. Yoga poses allow us the time and quiet space to acknowledge this relationship and we can feel that our bodies are secure and therefore able to relax. Through yoga we can also appreciate that all living things expanding and growing upwards counteract this downward pull of gravity. This understanding enables us to conduct each pose in accordance with the double action of stability and freedom. Yoga poses use the force of gravity to stabilise the base of the pose where our body parts meet the ground. This allows for the spinal column to elongate with the exhalation of the breath.

The Breath: Breathing is the foundation of all yoga poses and their counterpart, meditation. The simple act of following one's breath is the essence of mediation and serves to declutter the mind allowing the seeker a vision of a clearer truth. This can also apply to the student practicing yoga poses or asanas. I encourage students to allow the breath to dominate their being. It will act in two ways, to give energy for the stretch and enable peace for the mind. A student will inhale deeply through the nose and exhale through the mouth or the nose. I encourage them to think about filling their whole torso with breath and to feel the breath deep into the stomach. This is quite the contrast the shallow chest breathing that we doing in our daily breathing as we go about our business. Do this now as you read: inhale strongly through the nose filling your torso and then exhale through the mouth strongly. You will notice that the exhalation carries a strong power and a unique energy. This should be tapped into and harnessed during the stretches. Always move and deepen stretches on this powerful exhale. So for example if you decide to hold a pose for 8 breaths, on each exhale just push yourself slightly deeper into the posture. Move that arm, shoulder or leg just a bit more until you reach your edge, the point at which you have found maximum challenge and benefit. While you deepen each stretch use the calming repetition of the breath to follow and soothe away the tensions and struggles of the consciousness and also any discomfort and physical challenge offered by the posture itself. Utilising the power of this simple building block of life is simple. The easy act of following our breathing is empowering and illuminates our basic nature. We can leave behind the desires and chatter of our egos and access the calm and still essence of ourselves. This offers clarity of vision and the ability to make clearer decisions and better choices. All that is needed it the will to take out the time to understand it and use it to our advantage.

A student must always move into or further into a pose upon exhalation, and this movement is always a release away from the centre of the body into the periphery. There is an elongation of the body and an outward release of the body's tension. This is true even in poses that outwardly appear to be curled up such as Child's pose. The diaphragm contracts and relaxes as we breathe and is located inside of our torso across the bottom of the ribcage. At the back of the diaphragm are fibres, which extend down the front of the lumbar spine around our waist area. Here they meet the ilio psoas muscles. These also run along the front of the spine and then go down right through the back of the pelvis into the femurs at the top of the leg. These inner spinal muscles are vital for movement and postural alignment. They integrate the legs with the spine and affect the curve of the waist and the tilt of the pelvis. As you exhale these inner spinal muscles will release with the diaphragm allowing the curve at the back of the waist to lengthen. The abdominal muscles contract upon exhalation and balance this release at the back of the waist so that the lumbar spine lengthens and the pelvis drops down away from the waist when you are standing or sitting or in variations of these positions.

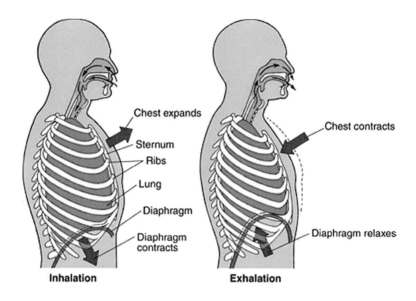

Inhalation — Exhalation

Chest expands
Sternum
Ribs
Lung
Diaphragm
Diaphragm contracts

Chest contracts
Diaphragm relaxes

This sequence of events allows for all students to benefit from a moment when the spine lengthens naturally with the exhalation and should allow them to achieve the yoga poses without effort. The exhalation releases tension and facilitates the dropping of the body or gravitating. All students need to take the quiet time to acknowledge their breathing patterns and feel the subtle shifts in their bodies that occur as a result of these changes to the breath. For this reason I often encourage a short breathing practice at the beginning of class so that all students can move away from unconscious breath patterns that dominate their pedestrian lives to deeper empowering breathing patterns that encourage movement. Bringing one's attention to breath brings you into the present moment and with time and practice quiet clear focus will emerge, this is your sanctuary.

The Spine: This is our central axis and fundamental not only to every physical movement but also mental movement as it houses the central nervous system that sends information to every part of the body. The work of yoga is to nurture and care for your spine and the other limbs and joints that stem from it. There is no pounding, impact or exertion that will leave you depleted soon after. You are caring for, servicing and recharging your vital structure in a way that no other form of exercise offers. This not only increases longevity of the spines complex functions but also facilitates comfort in whatever you are doing: standing at the supermarket checkout, sitting on an aeroplane or gardening. Practice of yoga enables movement with ease and comfort throughout the structure of your whole being.

The lowest curve of the spine is the composite bone of the sacrum formed of the five fixed vertebrae fused together with the rudimentary 'tail' of the coccyx beneath it. The sacrum forms the back of the pelvis or hip girdle as it fits between the two ilia bones, which flare out and curve round to meet the pubic symphasis at the front. The Ischia's bones or sitting bones, which we can feel under our buttocks when we sit, are the lowest part of the pelvis.

The pelvis and the sacrum are designed for strength, a bit above the sacrum the spine is made up of movable vertebrae with discs of cartilage between them to act as shock absorbers and make the spine elastic. The vertebrae are all slightly different from each other: the five lumbar vertebrae just above the sacrum are thick and strong. They carry much weight and fit in a way that allow only for slight restricted backbend or twisting movement. The twelve thoracic vertebrae, which carry the ribs, are more mobile. The ribcage needs to be able to stretch as well as protect as it carries the lungs and the heart. The seven cervical vertebrae in the neck are the smallest and lightest and have an extensive range of movement. At the back and sides of the vertebrae there are bony spines or processes protecting the spinal cord, which runs from the brain, and it's the main pathway of our nervous system.

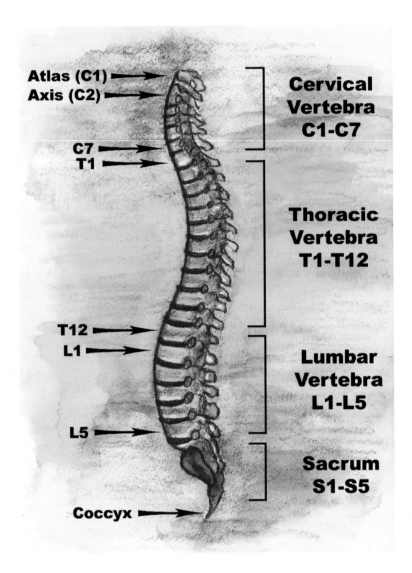

The spine needs to be strong and flexible and yoga using resistance bands can achieve both of these goals.

The bones of our skeleton are bound together by ligaments and enveloped by layers of muscles that constantly stretch and contract as we move. Our natural sense of balance ensures that our muscles continually tighten and release to hold us upright against the force of gravity that pulls us towards the centre of the earth. Habits of movement and restrictive positions can lead us to distort our posture. When this happens muscles that should be contracting and releasing have to tighten continually to hold a misaligned part of the body in place and the symmetry of our spinal curves become distorted. Yoga poses move the body in a myriad of different ways and directions. The poses allow the natural curves of the spine to elongate and readjust. As the spine releases in the yoga poses it will lengthen or elongate. This action divides the body below the waist. The lower half of the spine is pulled toward the ground and the upper half towards the sky. Through the poses we can not only regain postural balance but also stimulate the muscles, joints, circulation, digestion, nervous and endocrine systems that govern our health, general wellbeing and vitality.

CHAPTER 3

Preparation for Class and Warm-up

The Resistance Band

It is possible to purchase a resistance band to accommodate all levels of ability. They may be bought from a sports supply store or from an online supplier. They are light and portable so therefore easy to post. Chose a tubular band rather than a flat one and make sure that it has padded handles. Generally speaking the colour of the band indicates its intensity. Lighter colours provide less resistance and darker colours more intensity. They may be labelled on a scale of resistance. The leading brand that I use for classes manufactures bands ranging from a level one to a level three resistance. No standards exist between band manufacturers so check how the band feels if possible before purchase.

When you are using a resistance band for the first time pull it in opposing directions to test for resistance and durability. They should be replaced every couple of years on average but this will vary with the amount of usage.

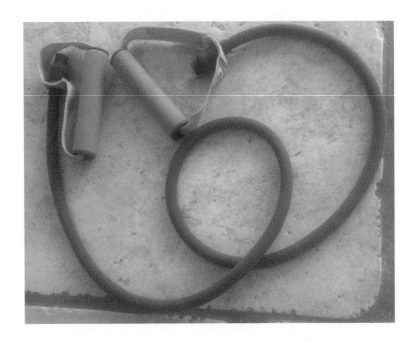

BEFORE THE CLASS BEGINS

At the start of each class I encourage students to connect with their breath. Doing so is a gateway between their hectic lives and the quiet break that the yoga class brings. The class is a 'mini holiday', an escape from pressures, problems and duties and an opportunity for recharging mind and body.

First I ask students to stand with their feet hip width apart.

When we stand, weight is transmitted down through our spines into our pelvis, through our hip joints to our feet. When the lower part of our body is grounded properly, the upper part of the body, including the mind, becomes light and agile. Energy is freed up. We learn to have our feet on the ground and in doing so realize our connection with the earth and we stretch and grow upwards towards the sky.

Next I ask students to drop their chins towards their collar bones. This is known as a chin lock in yoga circles. I use it here to rest the neck and eradicate tension in it before class begins. The seven vertebrae of the neck have an enormous burden to carry our heavy skull and are the most delicate and mobile part of the spine and therefore very vulnerable. Many students will come to class after a day at the office and consequently hold lots of tension in this area. I encourage students to release tension in the jaw when they have dropped their chins and be aware of any clenching movements. They should also relax their facial muscles. Then I ask them to follow their breath. The chin lock naturally lends to the slowing up of breathing and is a good position for the student to be still and simply observe the inhale and exhale. I try to encourage them to feel the natural movement of the belly as they breathe, let the back of their pelvis drop and arms and shoulders relax.

WARMING UP

Warming up involves moving the spine into the full range of positions available to it: Forward bending, backward bending, sidebending and twists.

Forward Bend

Standing straight take the resistance band in both hands and place it behind you. Next, bend forwards so that you drop the weight of your head towards the floor. The band will be behind your ankles, pull tight on it to deepen your forward bend. You will find that your arms will bend and that your head will naturally fall. Let the weight of the head deepen your forward bend and enjoy the benefits of inversion to the head. Blood will flow this way and stimulate your brain allowing for an improved alertness. The skin on your face will also benefit as the blood flow here will improve circulation and allow for rejuvenation of the skin. Acknowledge and appreciate these benefits everytime you allow this part of your body to enter inversion.

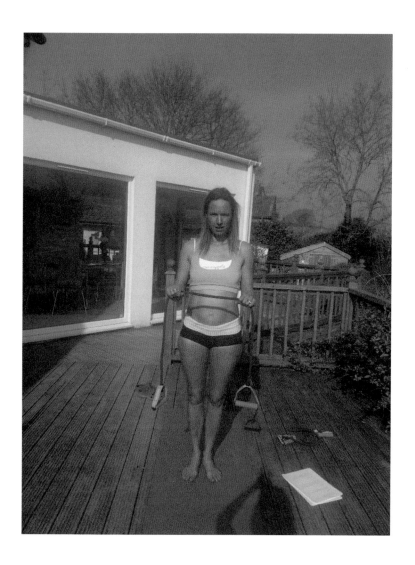

Before starting and folding forwards, stand tall on your mat. Your feet should have some space between them. Be aware of the weight being transmitted down your legs to your feet. Feel the contact of your heels with the mat. Stretch the band apart and feel the resistance that it offers.

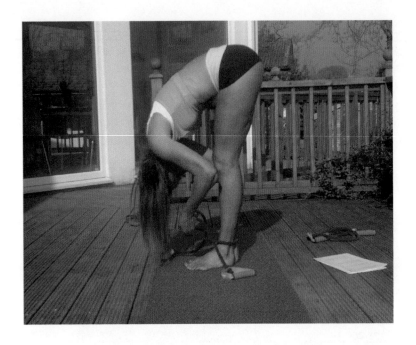

In the forward bend fold your torso over your legs and if necessary bend at the knees slightly to facilitate this. The position aims to target the lower back and not just the legs.

Forward Bend with a Twist

Standing legs wide apart hold the band in the air with two hands, drop forward and pull your hands away from each other. Now bring your opposite hand to the ankle and your other hand into the air. Repeat several times on each side.

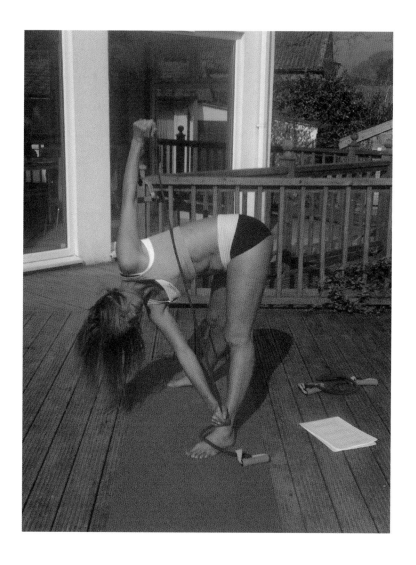

Here the top shoulder is key to a strong twist. Pull this shoulder back as far as possible whilst simultaneously pulling at the resistance band.

Backbend

Standing, hold the band in the air with two hands, and then pull the band behind you whilst simultaneously pulling your hands away from each other.

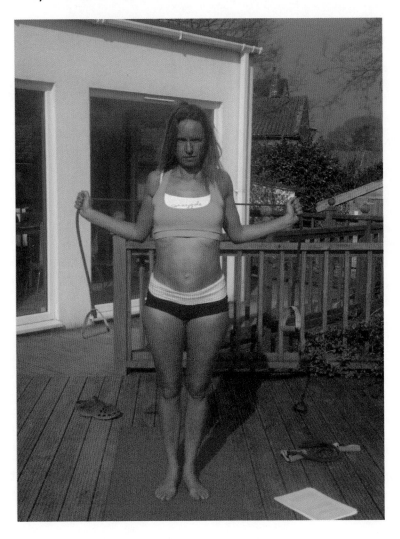

Backbend with a twist

Standing, hold the band in the air with two hands, you should be holding the middle third section of the band. Next, pull the band behind you whilst simultaneously pulling your hands away from each other. Then rotate your torso from left to right allowing your shoulders to turn behind you to lead your body into the twist.

As you rotate your shoulders from side to side sink heavily through both feet to keep yourself steady and balanced. Your shoulders are leading all the movement of your torso and you should twist them as far backwards and then forwards as possible. Visualise your healthy long spinal column twist right to left and imagine this movement realigning the vertebrae. The slight backbend that this movement offers will influence your thoracic (upper spine). This part of your back gets very little opportunity for movement during your pedestrian day. Feel the tension in the mid back release while simultaneously your shoulders move back and your chest opens. Most of us also stand with our shoulders rolled forwards without noticing so this backward movement helps to counteract this. Also moving the shoulders back will help you to open up your heart centre which is believed to govern your emotional well-being. Open your heart and rid yourself of any negative energy . Get everything "off of your chest".

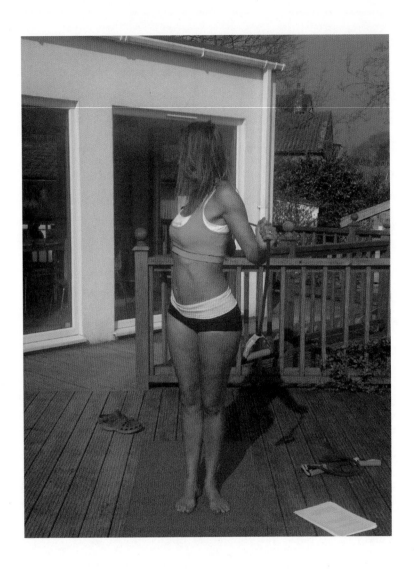

Notice how my head turns in this picture with my shoulders so that the cervical vertebrae in my neck also get the opportunity to benefit from the twist.

Backbend with legwork

Standing, turn your toes out sideways as far as possible, and then stand heels together. If you are thrown off balance take a wider stance. Next hold the band in the air with two hands and pull the band behind you whilst simultaneously pulling your hands away from each other. While you pull the band behind you tilt your tailbone forwards and bend your knees into a plia position. Working with a plia allows an understanding of pelvic awareness as the tailbone moves forwards and the hips mobilise. Many of our lives are stationary and we sit on chairs at desks and drive cars for a large part of our day. These positions detract from pelvic and general body awareness. We can forget our ability to move in this area and can indeed get away without moving the pelvis at all. Enjoy the control that you are capable of exerting over your pelvis as you bend the knees and tilt your tailbone forwards. Healthy pelvic movement is vital for all of our basic mobility so use yoga to regain a relationship with your pelvic area particularly if your job dictates a stationary position. When not in the work place you can extend this pelvic awareness by simply sitting on the floor or in a squatting position when circumstances allow.

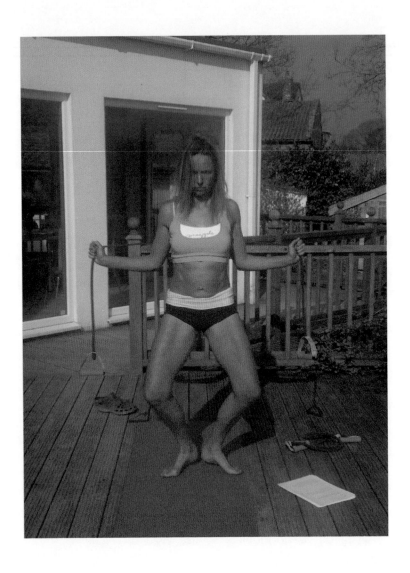

Try and keep your heels as close together as possible as this will
challenge the pelvis.

Sidebend

Standing, hold the band in the air and pull your hands away from each other. Keeping a straight stance bend to the right and lower the right hand. Then repeat on the left side. Do several times each side. We rarely open the sides of our spine, Enjoy!

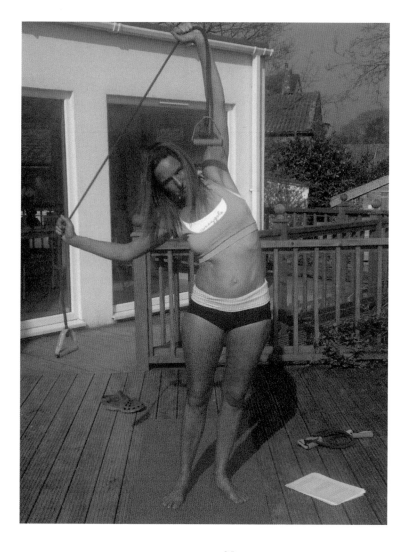

Twist

Stand with feet hip width apart. Place the band under the right foot and hold the handles together with both hands as high as possible keeping your arms straight. Swing your hands to the left taking care to turn the left shoulder as far as it will turn. Then swing the handles back to the right. Do this eight times and repeat the twists with the band under the left foot.

Twists are beneficial for all basic alignment of the spine. A standing twist requires strong anchoring in the feet but are suitable for all students and especially of value in pregnancy because the abdomen remains open and free. The shoulder is important in leading and deepening standing twists. Be aware of the position of the shoulder that is leading the twist and allow the shoulder to extend as far behind you as possible.

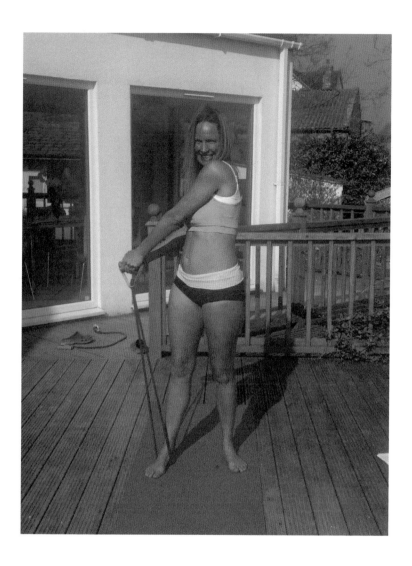

I am looking forward here to smile at the camera! Try to keep your gaze during the exercise in line with the movement of the shoulder so that the top of your spine (the neck) can also twist.

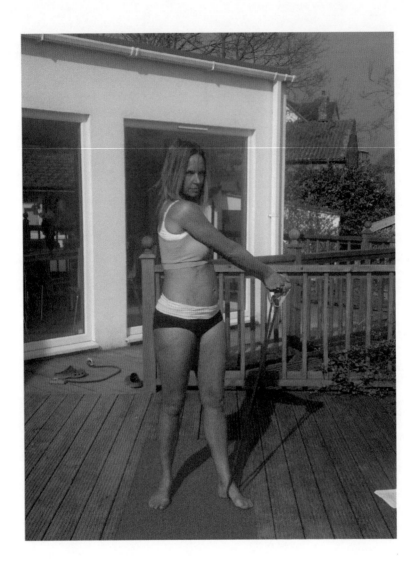

Keep a wide stance with your feet for balance and stability and focus on the feeling of the ground beneath your feet. If you do this your feet will sink firmly downwards supporting the movement of the rest of your body.

CHAPTER 4

Balances

We all lose our ability to balance as we age. Regular practice can counteract this process. Balances also aid concentration as they force us to think and concentrate in the present moment. Think of your standing foot as growing roots and grow them down below the big toe, little toe and heel. Gaze at something stationary to help settle the mind but don't stare. Maintain a distant gaze, breath into the abdomen and enjoy the simplicity of the present moment.

The Dancer

Standing on the right leg loop the band under the left foot just in front of the toe area. Bend the left knee and let the band stretch behind your body holding the handles above your head. First keep the knees together and feel the stretch to your left quad and the backbend to the lower back. For more challenge start to move the handles of the band forward as you let your bent leg rise higher into the air. Cast your gaze at something stationary and enjoy some deep breaths. Firmly plant your standing foot on the ground, let gravity assist you and feel the three points of the foot (under the big toe, little toe and heel) sink downwards as your upper body stretches upwards. Stay for a minimum of eight deep breaths and then repeat on the other side of the body.

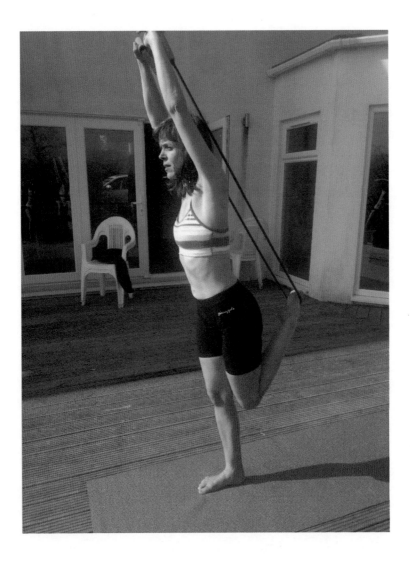

Using a resistance band as an aid to support a student in this classical yoga pose allows their spine to remain straight. In the classical yoga pose most students will reach behind them to grab their foot, which puts their spine out of line. Holding the handles of the band above the head allows the spine to be straight and elongated.

Warrior 3

This balance is similar to the Dancer pose except that the raised leg remains straight and the aim is to get the body straight and parallel to the floor. Start by standing on the right foot and loop the band under the left foot. Gently raise the left leg into the air and hold one handle of each band in each of your hands. Tilt the torso forwards and aim to be parallel to the floor from your hands to your raised left foot. The toes of this raised foot should point downwards. For increased balance you may experiment with slightly bending the standing leg. Cast your distant gaze at a stationary spot. Maintain a deep and easy breathing pattern for a minimum of eight breaths. Now switch sides, your left leg is your standing leg.

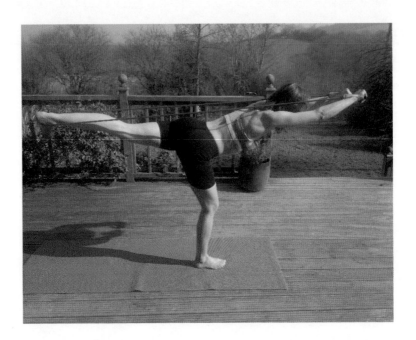

Notice the straight line between the student's back foot and hands. Using the band helps to keeps both high as dropping the raised leg or arms can be a common mistake in Warrior 3 pose and is not possible with the aid of the resistance band.

Tree pose

Start by standing straight. Your right foot will be your standing foot. Put your left foot into the handle of the resistance band. Bend your left leg and pull your left foot as high as you can on the front of the right thigh. Turn your left knee downwards.

You should be holding the resistance band with your right hand and should now reach your left hand into the air. If you prefer you may hold the resistance band in both hands. As you exhale, press down firmly on the outer heel of your standing leg to strengthen and stabilize your pelvis. Dropping the bent knee down away from your hip will help to lengthen your waist. Stay in this pose for a minimum of 8 breaths maintaining a relaxed gaze. Repeat on the other side.

Using the resistance band to assist the student with this popular classical yoga pose allows the band to support the student's knee fully. Many students find that their foot slips when they fix it to the inside of the standing leg as the classical yoga pose dictates. This is exacerbated by the type of leg wear that in used. Synthetic materials can also make gripping with the sole of the foot to the standing leg difficult.

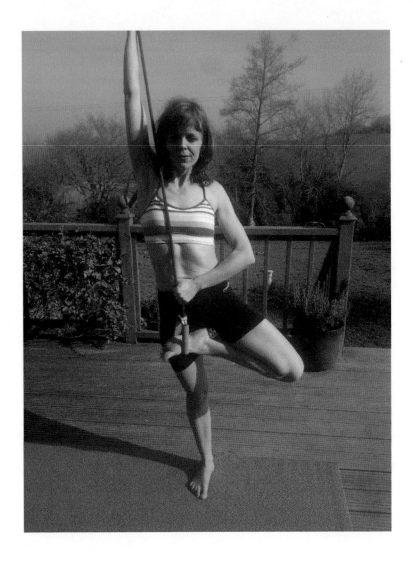

The resistance band allows the hip to open while supporting the student's foot. The band also follows the length of the spine encouraging a straight line of elongation.

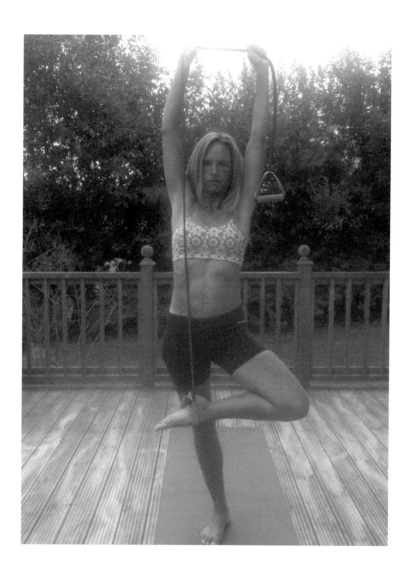

In this example both hands are raised above the head. This will stretch the torso and spine while allowing the hip of the bent leg to open.

Big toe Pose

Start by standing straight. Your right foot will be your standing foot. Sink this foot downwards and feel your foots firm and steady contact with the ground. Put your left foot through the handle of the resistance band. Raise the leg foot into the air in front of your body holding the resistance band in both hands fairly close to the handle. Next, holding the resistance band in your left hand allow the left foot to travel to the left, aiming to keep your left leg parallel to the ground. Stretch your right hand out to the side. Next bring the leg back to the front of the body and taking the band in the right hand allow the leg to travel as far to the right as it will go aiming to keep it parallel to the floor. Repeat on the other side.

Using a resistance band to assist this yoga classic allows for a deeper extension in the elevated leg. In the traditional asana students are required to hold the big toe but this is often a difficult task especially for those students with lovely long legs. The band will alleviate this issue, making the pose accessible for all body shapes.

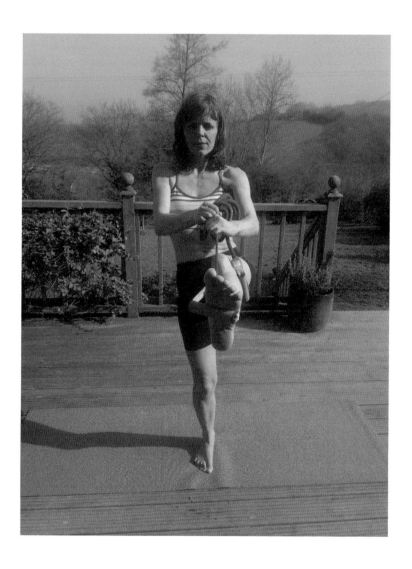

Keep a firm and strong hold on your resistance band while simultaneously 'growing roots' into the ground with your standing foot.

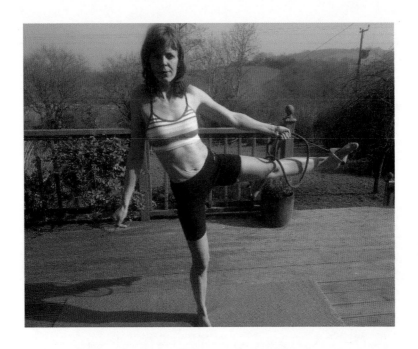

Extend the elevated leg as far out to the side as possible. This will challenge and open your hip. Aim to keep the elevated leg parallel to the ground. If you feel wobbly, a slight bend to the standing leg can often be helpful. Relax your shoulders and stand and take deep breaths in this posture. Keep your mind in the present moment and be in a state of quiet calm. Your body will respond with a steady and calm balance.

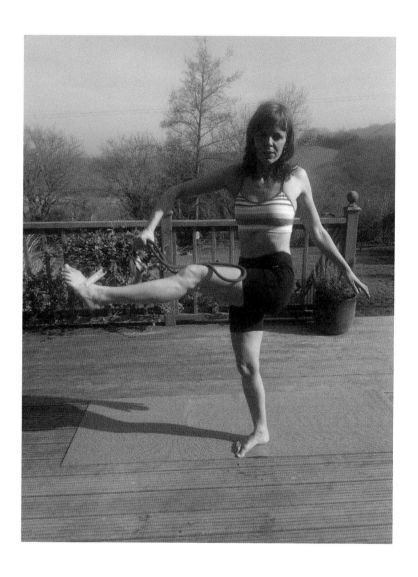

This position allows for a pelvic twist in the opposite direction. If you feel very ambitious you may fold your torso over the elevated leg bringing your head to the elevated knee before finally exiting the posture and repeating on the other side.

Gate Pose as a balance

Kneel with your thighs off of the ground. Extend your right leg out to the side keeping the toes of the right foot pointing forwards. Place the handle of the resistance band under the right foot. Holding the resistance band in the centre of its length pull on the band with both hands and simultaneously lean your torso towards your right foot. Experience the side bend to the waist and hold for several breaths. Next elevate the right leg so that it is parallel to the floor. Turn the toes of the right foot downwards. Place your left hand next to your left knee to support you in this balance and hold the band in its centre with your right hand. Stay in this balance for several breaths. If you wish to be active in this balance and challenge the muscles of the elevated leg further you may raise and lower the right leg allowing the toes to touch the floor and each time bringing the leg back to reach a position that is parallel to the floor. Repeat on the other side.

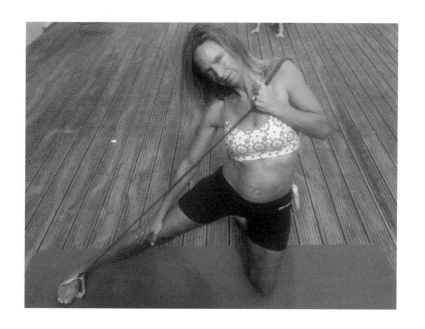

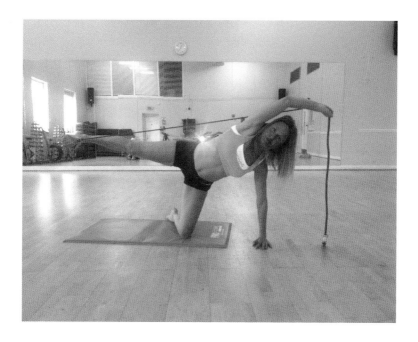

CHAPTER 5

Standing Poses

The Warriors

Fierce Warrior!

The Warrior in your heart says to stand your ground

Feel the survival of a thousand years of ancestors in your muscles and your blood

You have all the support that you need in your bones....

As the name implies, the Warrior poses are based on fighting stances, and are similar to those in the martial arts. The power of these poses is in the legs and pelvis. Students should think off their back standing foot as a strong anchor. The upper body remains light and free.

Warrior One

Start in standing and then step forward with your right leg. Exhaling bend your right knee. Place the band under the left back foot. The further apart your feet are the harder your legs will have to work, therefore choose a stance to match your energy levels. If you feel at all wobbly or off balance then widen your stance. The toes of your back foot should be facing forward the same way as your front foot. This will keep the pelvis facing forward. The position of the pelvis is important. If the back foot toes are turned out the pelvis turns to the side (as it should be in Warrior two pose) and this may make the sacrum vulnerable to shearing. Exhaling bring the handles into the air with both hands. Keep the line of the spine vertical and drop weight through the pelvis on the exhalation. The whole spine is encouraged to stretch and elongate as the arms lead the stretch above the head.

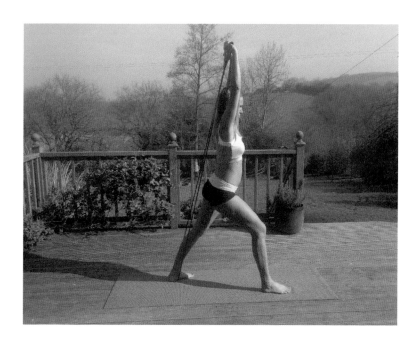

The picture above demonstrates how the spine follows the length of the resistance band. The band encourages elongation as the resistance of the rubber pushes the stretch higher than the student would likely reach with their hands alone.

Remember that your back foot anchors the posture. You should continue to ground or depress through this foot using the force of gravity to assist you. In doing so the rest of your body is encouraged to rise upwards away from this anchorage and find maximum expansion.

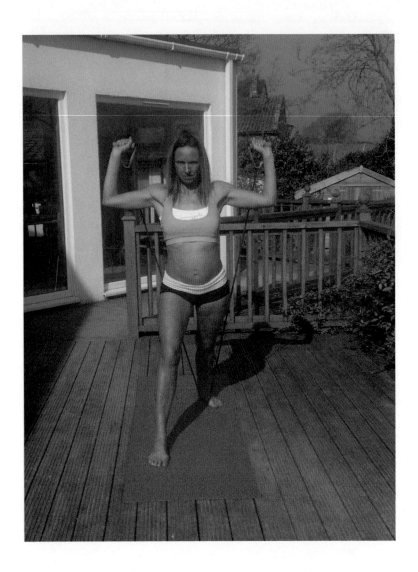

If you wish to engage in a more dynamic variation then raise
and lower your arms so that arms maintain an L shape on
lowering. When you have done a minimum of 8 breaths or 8
arm raises then switch sides.

Warrior Two

Start by standing straight. Step your right foot forward and place the band under the back left foot. Place your weight on your back foot. The back foot should be strongly depressed just as in Warrior One pose and anchors the posture. However, the back foot is more turned out in this pose than in Warrior One and you may let it be parallel to the back edge of your yoga mat. Here your pelvis should face sideways rather than forwards. Holding the handles of the band in each hand bring both arms up sideways. Pull the hands as high as possible against the resistance of the band. Feel the power of this stretch through your arms and across your mid spine. Using the resistance band for this yoga classic, incorporates upper body strengthening and conditioning into a yoga pose that classically focused on the lower body. If you like an active variation you may move the hands in this pose to promote a twist. Move your front and back hands clockwise. Hold for a minimum of eight breaths or twists. Switch sides. To do the active twist variation with your left foot forwards move both handles in an anti-clockwise position.

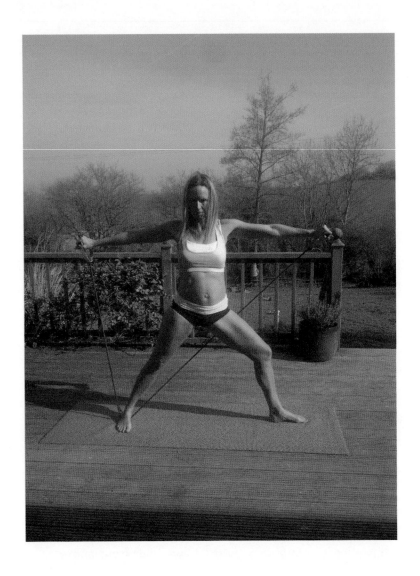

Adjust the distance between your feet according to your energy levels.

The further your feet are apart the more challenge to the muscles in the

legs. Make sure your back foot is parallel to the back of the mat, as this

will keep the alignment of the pelvis healthy without shearing. Enjoy the power of this pose in both the upper and lower body.

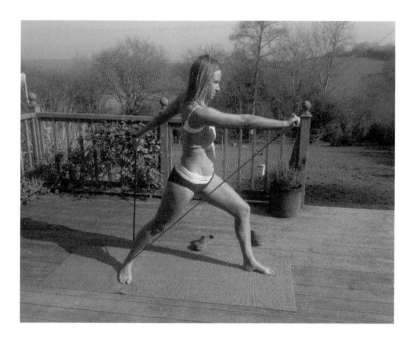

This picture demonstrates the dynamic variation. Here I swing my arms forwards and backwards and this promotes a strong twist for the mid or thoracic spine. I am a fan of promoting twisting in classical yoga positions whenever viable. Twists eliminate stiffness, conquer injury and are key to the prevention of general spine deterioration.

Chair Pose

This is a simple pose that allows your legs to grow strong. It is also useful to practice pelvic awareness. Start by standing straight with your feet hip width apart. Stand on your resistance band and then cross the band over and hold the handles. Bring your arms in front of you. Next, bend your knees and sit in the seat of your imaginary chair. Visualise the chair that you desire and let your pelvis drop into this soft and comfortable chair. Breathe deeply and steadily. You may stay in this chair as long as you wish and as long as it is comfortable. To exit the pose, exhale press on your feet and start to straighten your legs. As you come up tilt your pelvis forwards. This is done simply by tucking in your pelvis and adjusting your tailbone so that it moves forwards. When you return to standing, release the pelvic tilt. Continue to sit in your chair and return to standing. Repeat this action a minimum of eight times.

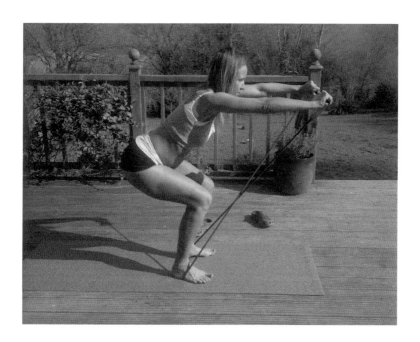

Using the resistance band to assist with this yoga classic allows the student a great deal of extra support in the posture. Rather than simply being suspended in space and reaching forwards, as Chair is classically taught the student here is able to push away from the feet with the band. This offers support to the pelvis and enables any student to gain a deeper seat in their chair than they could otherwise unassisted by the band.

CHAPTER 6

Poses for a Strong Core

The Boat

The following poses aim to build abdominal muscles, which serve as protection for the lower spine.

Warming up the abdominals

Wrap the band around the feet by passing it across the top of the feet and then under both feet, bringing both handles inside the foot. Take the handles in two hands and lie down holding the handles at rib level. Your head and shoulders are flat to the ground. Now slowly raise your legs so that they become perpendicular to the body. Your lower back upwards is flushed to the ground. Your feet are flexed and you should push through the heels as you come up. Then slowly lower both feet back to the ground keeping the handles at rib level. Repeat for three sets of eight. To modify for ease you can bend slightly at the knees.

To assure lower back support, keep it firmly in contact with the ground during the whole of this exercise and don't let it lose this contact when the legs swing up off the floor.

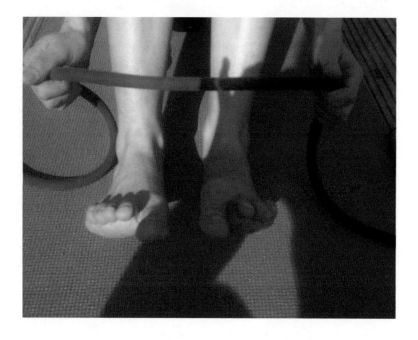

Notice in the below picture how the resistance band first passes across the top of the student's feet and then the handles are passed through the inside edges of the foot. The result is a firm and slip free grip for the band onto both feet.

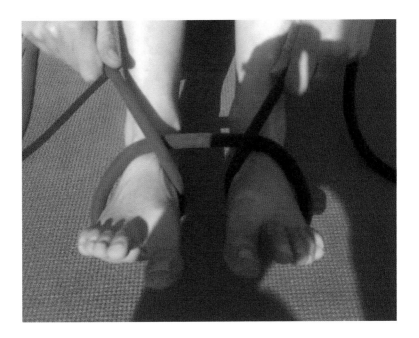

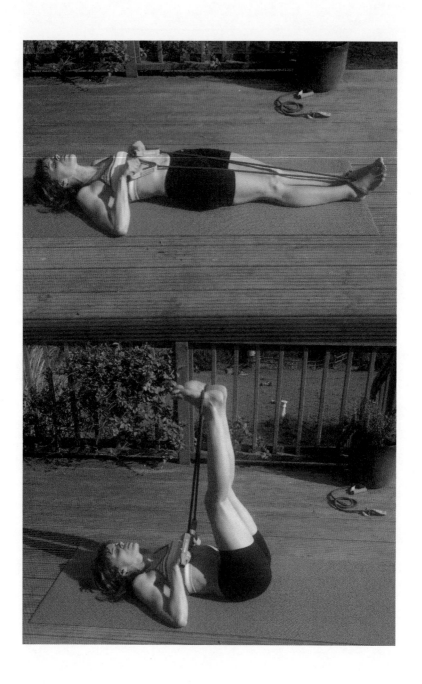

Boat Pose

Sitting with your legs slightly bent pass the band across the top of your feet and under the feet, then pass the handles between the inside edges of both feet and hold them at chest height. Straighten your legs and hold your body into a V position. Drop your shoulders back and away from your ears. Allow your back to assume a straight diagonal line. If this position causes any lower back discomfort modify by bringing your upper and lower back flat to the floor and raise the legs into the air using the floor for support. After practice, your abdominals will strengthen and you will be able to adopt boat in the sitting position. If you are in sitting boat you may make the pose more challenging by lowering the upper body and the legs so that the body now resembles a very wide V shape.

Keep the handles of the resistance band tight to the chest during this pose and feel the support that the band gives you to maintain this posture. Using the resistance band allows the student to stay in boat pose for far longer and keep the spine straighter than if the pose was unassisted by the band.

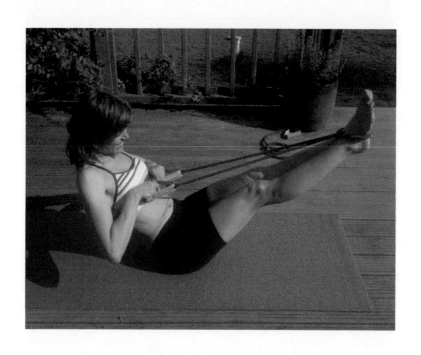

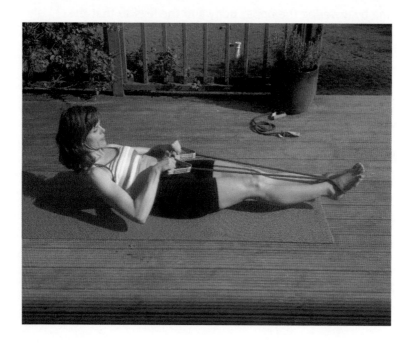

Boat Modification: Boat and Fish pose

Sitting with your legs slightly bent pass the band across the top of your feet and under the feet, then pass handles between the inside edges of the feet and hold them at chest height. Lowering yourself to the floor rest on your elbows and on the spot just behind the top of your head. Experience the stretch to the neck. Fish pose is thought to be beneficial to the thyroid as it provides a stretch to this area. Next bring your feet into boat position feet into the air. They should be just short of a ninety-degree angle. If you enjoy activity you may raise and lower the legs in a slow and controlled manner keeping the handles of the band at chest level.

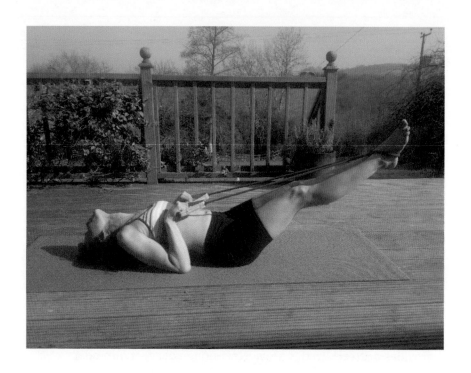

CHAPTER 7

Backbends

Back bending poses are considered to be energetic, energising, dynamic, extroverted and stimulating as the whole front of the spine opens. The neck and lower back are easier to bend in this fashion so students need to focus with extra attention on their stiffer upper backs or thoracic spine. The whole spine should move as this will prevent jarring, overstretching and injury.

Lotus Pose

Lie on your stomach and stretch your fingertips away from your toes. Depress the pelvic area and think of the pelvis as a heavy base for the rest of the pose. Take the resistance band in two hands so that there is a third of the band between your hands. On an inhalation pull the band behind your back as you lift your chest and legs from the ground simultaneously. Exhaling bring your body back to the ground. Repeat this action several times. The breathing pattern here is reversed from most poses as the movement into the position is on an inhalation instead of the exhalation. This is because the inhalation here encourages the chest to open and expand whereas an exhalation lends itself to a natural sinking of the chest. You may also rock gently side to side in the pose when you are in the elevated position, as this will encourage further movement in the upper spine. On completion rest on your stomach sinking the whole body into the mat on the exhalation. Rest for several breaths.

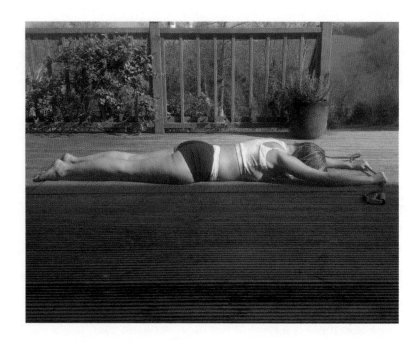

Using a resistance band for the locust pose enables any student to exaggerate the backbend in the upper spine. The band fixes the arms in a position to promote this strong backbend in a way that would not be possible without the aid of the resistance band.

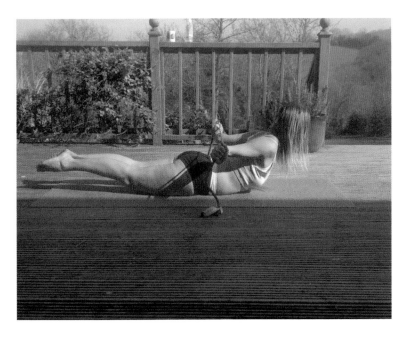

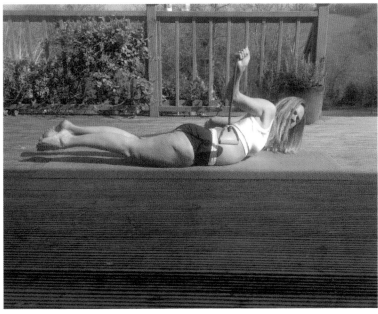

Bow

Like locust pose, bow pose is also good for opening the upper chest and the front of the shoulders. Sitting, place the band across the top of the feet and then allow the handles of the resistance band to pass inside the inner edges of the feet. Next, lie on your stomach and hold the handles of the band outside of each leg.   Then push the handles of the resistance bands in front of your body straightening your arms as if to punch the air. Simultaneously use the resistance bands to raise your feet into the air. Move into the pose on the inhalation lifting your chest off the ground and raising your feet. Imagine that you are trying to stretch them out straight into the air but keep them parallel and don't allow your knees to drop too far apart, bring them as close together as you can. Draw your tailbone and sitting bones under, depressing the pelvis to the ground in a similar fashion to locust pose. Let your head follow the movement of the spine and breathe deeply expanding the chest and pulling the shoulders back on the inhalation. Use the exhalation to depress or ground the pelvis.

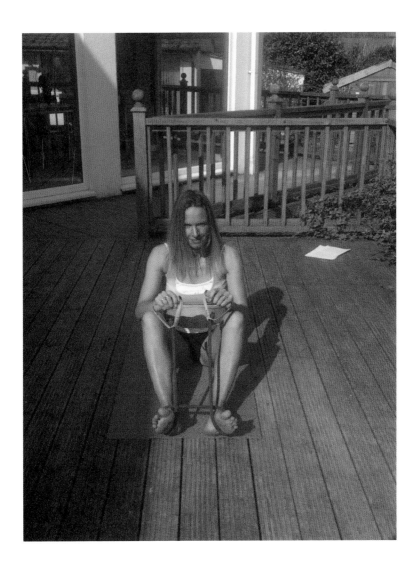

Many students find it hard to reach for their feet as required in the traditional bow pose. Using the resistance band eliminates this problem while encouraging a strong backbend for the whole spine. In the traditional pose the backbend is very much focused on the lower back only.

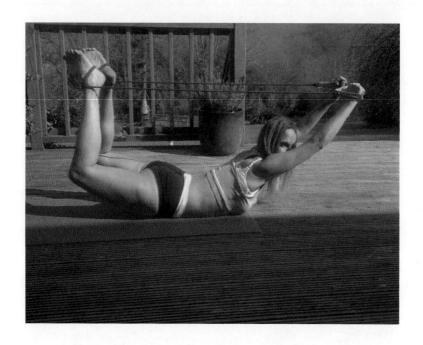

Modification

Some students may find that the method of wrapping the band around both of the feet to be cumbersome in the Bow pose. If this is the case for you simply lie on your stomach and bend the knees, then place the band across the tops of both feet without wrapping it. Pull the handles in front of you as you raise your feet high into the air and expand through your chest as you move into the pose.

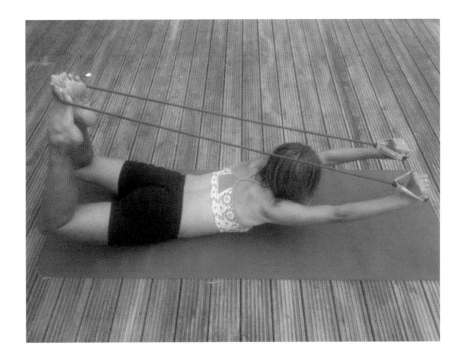

Camel

Start in a kneeling position and then take the resistance band
and place under your feet so that it lies between the tops of
your feet and the floor. Hold the hands of the band in both
hands. Keep your thighs as vertical as you can and imagine that
someone is holding a rope around your pelvis and it pulling it
forward. Do not collapse backwards. On an exhalation, pull
both handles of the bands into the air straightening your arms
as you do so. Looking up at the handles breathe deeply,
encouraging breath into the belly. Keep the back of your neck

long. Bend your arms to release from this pose and then repeat several times.

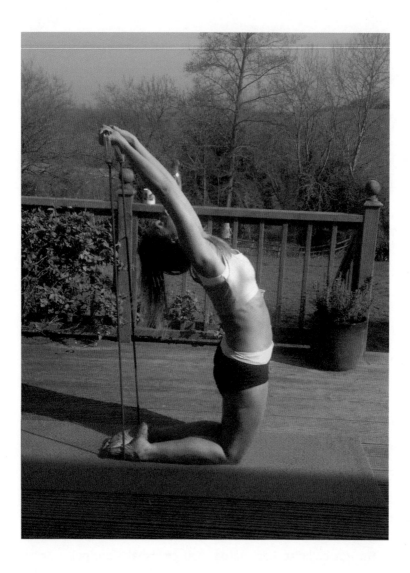

Keep your gaze directed at the handles of the resistance band when practicing Camel. This will ensure that your neck also is engaged in a back bending stretch.

Bridge

Start by lying on your back with your knees bent and your feet on the floor hip width apart. Place the resistance band under your feet and hold the handles in both hands. Depress your inner feet into the floor and imagine that you are carrying a football between your knees. Exhaling straighten your arms behind you and lift your pelvis off the floor. Drop your chin towards your collarbone. Stay in the pose breathing deeply and raising the pelvis on the exhalation. Relax your arms and slowly peel the spine back down to the floor working down through the vertebra from the neck to the waist. When ready, on an exhalation enter the pose again and repeat several times.

Using the resistance band to assist with this classical chest opener promotes a much stronger elongation throughout the whole spinal column. This is because the hands pull the spine away from the tailbone against the strong resistance the band offers.

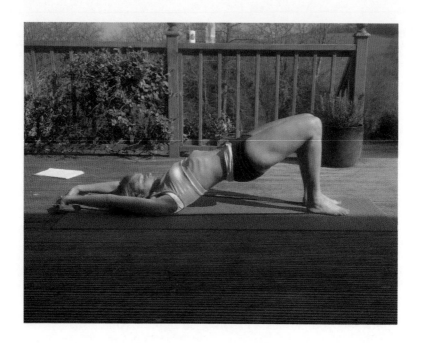

Hero

This pose involves sitting and then lying back between your heels and offers an intense stretch for the leg and joints of the leg. Start by kneeling with your knees hip width apart and your feet wider apart than your hips. Bend your knees and sit down between your heels. Next, pass the resistance band under the tops of your feet. Hold the handles of the band. Drop back onto your elbows and then if you can drop onto the top of your head and straighten your hands pulling the handles of the resistance band behind you. Breathing deeply hold the pose for a several breaths and exit the pose slowly.

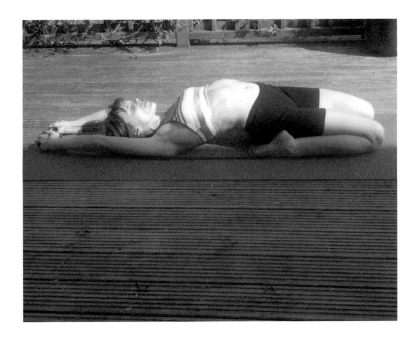

Modification

This pose may be very difficult for some students as the stretch in the thigh muscles and the ligaments around the knees is intense. If this is the case modify by bending only one leg. Loop the resistance band under the foot of this leg and keep the other leg straight out in front of you. Lie back pulling both handles of the resistance band behind you.

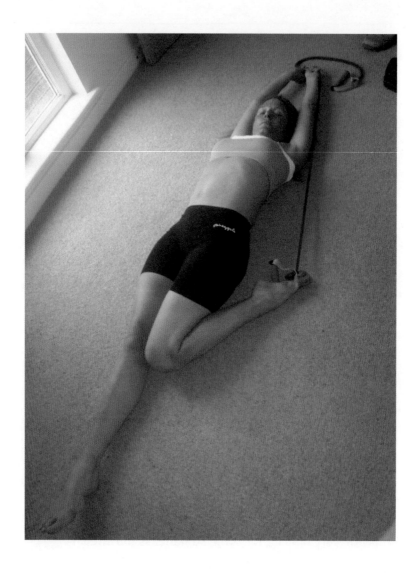

In a similar fashion to the bridge pose, here the resistance band promotes a deeper elongation of the spine as the arms stretch behind the body against the resistance of the rubber tubing.

Variation- Heron

Start by sitting with your legs straight. Bend one leg back as in Hero's Pose. Put the resistance band around the bottom of the straight leg foot and bring the foot into the air. Straighten your lifted leg up towards the ceiling with the assistance of the resistance band. Your leg and spine will form a "V" shape. Breathe deeply and on the exhalation your spine and lifted leg will stretch and elongate. Depress or ground your outer hips downwards. Your chest should lift upwards. Pull the elevated thigh towards your torso. The closer you can get it to your belly and chest, the better. Stay for several breaths before switching sides.

Using the resistance band to assist in this posture eliminates the need to reach for the elevated foot. This allows the student to focus upon grounding or depressing the pelvis as the foot and chest lift upwards without strain or difficulty. As the student becomes more practiced, the spine straightens as the chest continues to lift forwards.

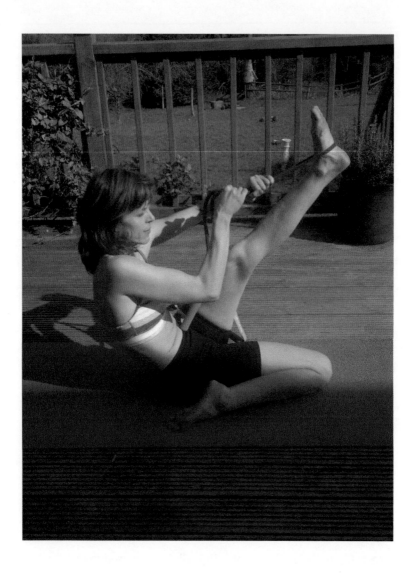

Notice how the resistance band helps to promote a strong and stable foundation for this pose as it eliminates the struggle to reach for and hold onto the foot, which is a difficult challenge, particularly for yoga novices.

CHAPTER 8

Forward Bends

Forward bends are introspective and nurturing poses. Make these postures your focus during times of illness, weakness and mental challenges. Rest into them for long periods and allow yourself the quiet refuge offered by them allowing your body to recuperate.

Basic Sitting Forward Bend

Start by sitting on the floor with both legs straight out in front of you. Next, place the resistance band under your feet. Holding the band with each hand, exhale and drop the back of your pelvis and elongate your spine to stretch forward. Aim to fold your stomach over your thighs. If this is difficult at first simply bend the legs in order to fold your stomach over the thighs. To avoid strain in the neck your head should just be low and rested. Stay forward as long as desirable breathing deeply and exit on an exhalation.

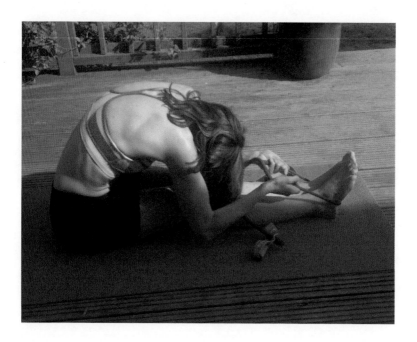

Sitting with legs wide Forward Bend

Start by sitting with your legs wide apart. Place the resistance band under the feet and hold both handles in each hand. Pull your torso forwards over the space between the legs. Breathe deeply pulling more forwards into the pose on the exhalation. This pose stretches the inner thighs and the hamstrings. For a variation turn to the right and loop the resistance band over the right foot. On an exhalation, stretch forward over your right leg while depressing through your left sitting bone. Stay forward breathing deeply and moving forwards into the pose on the exhalation. When ready release and repeat on the other side.

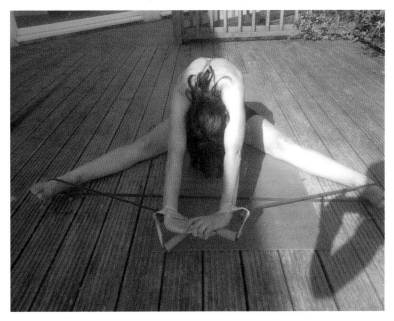

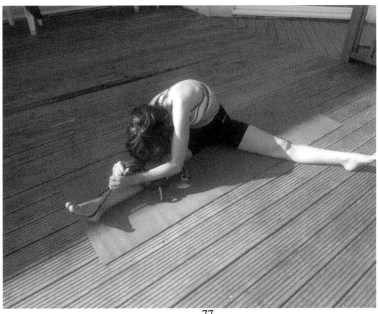

Many students find forward bending from a seated position particularly challenging. Using a resistance band helps them to achieve a deeper than otherwise possible pose. This is because they can anchor their sitting bones as they pull themselves forwards with the assistance of the band. Without the band many student feel 'stuck', particularly in the legs wide variation of the forward bend. The band allows for continuous deepening within the postures.

Sitting Forward Bend with one leg Bent

Start by sitting with your legs straight. Bend one leg and place your heel on the inside of the straight leg as high up the leg as possible. Put the resistance band under the foot of the straight leg. Pull yourself over the straight leg with the assistance of the band. As you exhale let your bent leg release away from your hip and drop towards the floor. Keep the bent knee as far away from the straight leg as possible. Deepen the stretch on the exhalation by dropping the pelvis and bent knee while keeping your spine and straight leg long. Repeat on the other side.

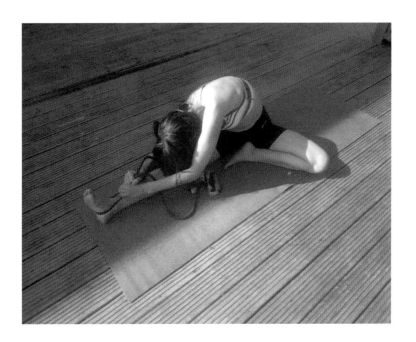

Variation

Start by sitting with your legs straight. Bend the right leg and place the heel on the inside of the left leg as high as possible up this leg. Pull the resistance band under the left foot. Hold the band in the left hand and settle the left elbow to the ground inside of the left leg. Bring your right arm into the air and stretch your right hand towards your left big toe. Catch it if you can, although if you can't, simply stretch towards this toe. As you exhale let your bent leg release way from your hip and drop towards the floor. Experience the deep stretch to your right side. Stay in the pose deepening the stretch on the exhalation.

When you are ready switch sides.

This pose offers the student a strong sidebend which is of great value to the spine because sidebending rarely arises in our everyday movement. Therefore, stretches which open the side of the spine to promote space and flexibility, are of special value. Using the resistance band eliminates the need to hold onto the foot which many students find difficult.

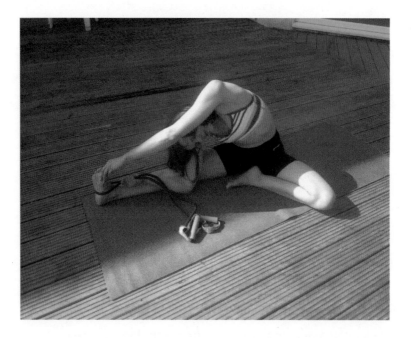

Half Lotus Forward Bend

Start by sitting with your legs straight. Next bend one leg and place your foot on the opposite thigh. Place the resistance band under the foot of the straight leg. Using the resistance band to help pull yourself forward over the straight leg, breathing deeply and elongating the spine and sinking the torso forwards on the exhalation. Do not put strain on the knee or ankle of the bent leg. If this happens move the foot of the bent leg down towards the thigh. Stay in the pose for several breaths and then come up and repeat on the other side.

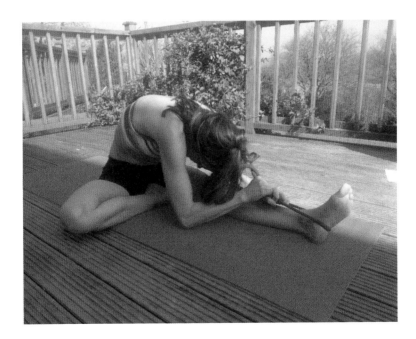

Plough Pose

Sitting, place the resistance band across the top of your foot and pass the handles through the inside edges of both feet. Hold the handles of the resistance band in both hands and roll backwards as if performing a half somersault. Allow your feet to drop to or towards the space behind your head. Let them travel as far as they will drop. Next, straighten your arms away from your head. This encourages your neck, shoulders and spine to elongate. Hold for several breaths. Plough is a wonderful forward bend as gravity helps to fold the spine forwards in such a way that sitting forward bend can't accommodate. Although is the same as a sitting forward bend only in its inverted form the corresponding stretch offered will always be deeper.

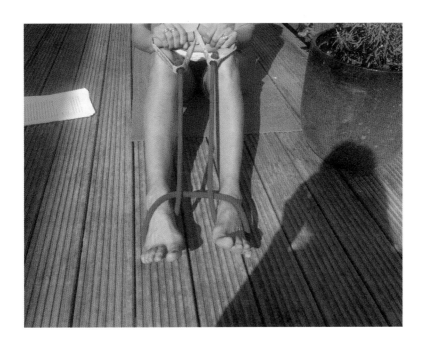

For the Plough pose we are once again using the wrap method to secure the feet. The band is passes across the top of the foot, then both handles are passed through the inside edges of the feet. This wrapping method results in a secure non-slip grip of both feet.

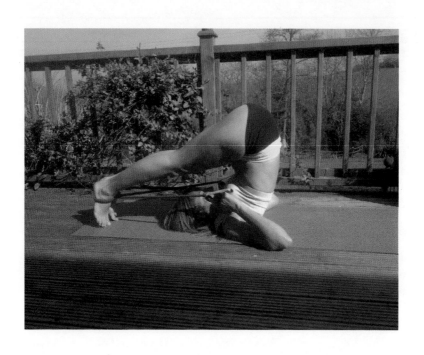

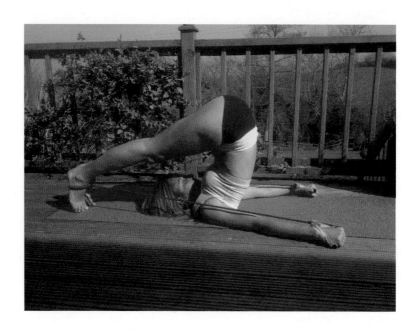

Childs's Pose

Sit on your heels and place the resistance band under your feet. Hold the handles in both hands. Bend forward and rest your arms and head on the floor stretching your arms out straight in front of you. Breathe deeply and on the exhalation let your hips drop back towards your heels. Simultaneously reach further forward with your arms and let your head and shoulders drop.

Child's pose is unique in its simplicity and gives special relief for those with lower back trouble. Accessible to all, it promotes a strong but gentle forward bend for the lower back while simultaneously allowing the hips to open. Using the resistance band to assist with this pose allows for a deep spinal elongation as the hands reach away from the pelvis stretching the spine forward. The resistance offered by the rubber tubing makes this stretch much stronger.

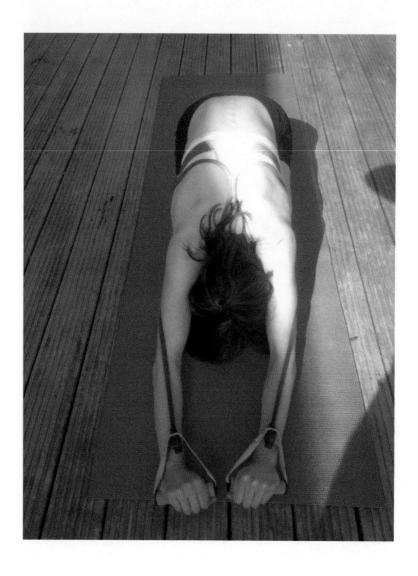

In this picture the student's spine is elongated through the arms
pushing forward against the resistance of the band. This simple pose
also offers rest and rejuvenation for the whole body while the lower
back and pelvis opens and releases tension.

CHAPTER 9

Twists

Sage's Twist

Start by sitting on the floor with both legs straight. Next bend your right leg and place your right foot upon the floor as close as possible to your right sitting bone. Rotate your torso to the left. Hold the resistance band in your right hand and then place this hand inside of the thigh of the right leg. Wrap your arm around your right leg. Next bend your left arm and reach this arm behind you to take the resistance band close to your right hand. Hug your right knee close to your body keeping as little space as possible between your thigh and ribs. Depress weight into the inside edge of the right foot and keep the shin of this leg vertical. Breathe deeply and upon the exhalation press down with your right foot and depress the pelvis using gravity to encourage your body to twist and your hip to release. Turn your head to the left and stretch out your left leg in front of you. Breathe deeply several breaths and then release the resistance band and repeat on the other side.

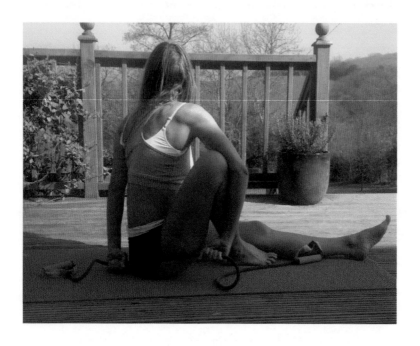

Half Lotus Twist

Sit with your legs straight out in front of you. Take your left foot and let it rest high on your right thigh. Next place your left foot in one of the handles of the resistance band. With your right hand tug the resistance band to the right and behind of you, rotating your right shoulder back as you do this. Deeply breathe pulling the left foot high on the right leg and turning your shoulder to promote the twist. Drop your sitting bones on the exhalation. Stay for several breaths and then switch sides.

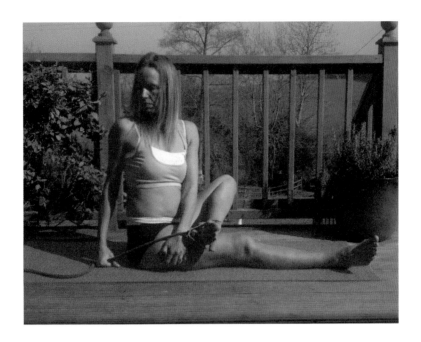

Using the resistance band to assist with this sitting twist enables the student to have a firm grip on their foot which opens the hip nicely without slouching in the spine. Sitting with the spine tall and straight allows the maximum benefit to the spine's alignment.

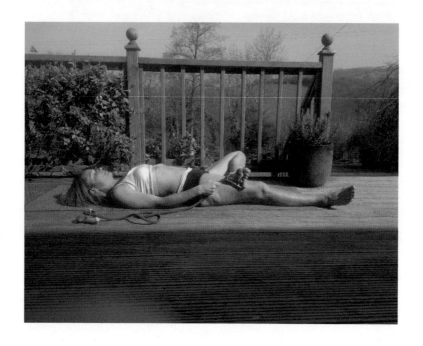

Finish by laying back in the half lotus pose. Relax and pull your foot high. On the exhalation sink you weight downwards allowing your body to feel heavy and relaxed. Focus particularly on depressing through the bent knee to open up the pelvis. Stay as long as you wish and then switch sides.

Laying Twist

Lay flat on the floor with legs straight and put the resistance band under your right foot. Raise the foot into the air holding the resistance band in both hands. Next hold both sides of the resistance band with your left hand and allow the foot to travel to the left. Keep your shoulders sinking into the floor. Let your belly button face the ceiling ensuring that your torso does not roll to the left. Pull the foot towards the shoulder and don't worry if it doesn't reach the ground. When your right foot has travelled as far left as it can go hold the pose and breathe deeply into your abdomen sinking your shoulders on the exhalation. When finished let the right foot travel back to being directly above your body. Take the band in the right hand and let the right foot travel to the right to give the right inner leg and groin a stretch. Hold this stretch and then change to the left foot and repeat the whole sequence.

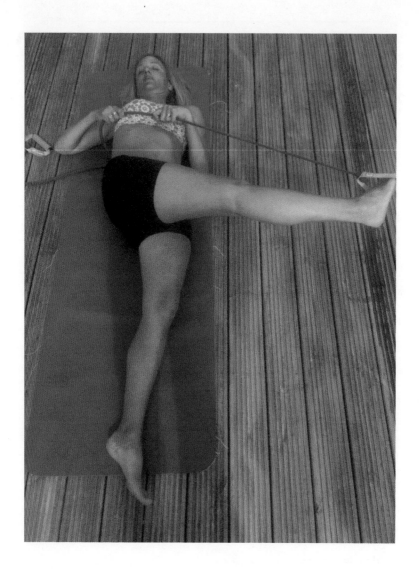

Using a resistance band for this stretch enables the student to sink into a deep lower spine twist that also opens the pelvis. There is no strain or pressure to hold the leg or foot and the student may remain relaxed and heavy throughout the upper body.

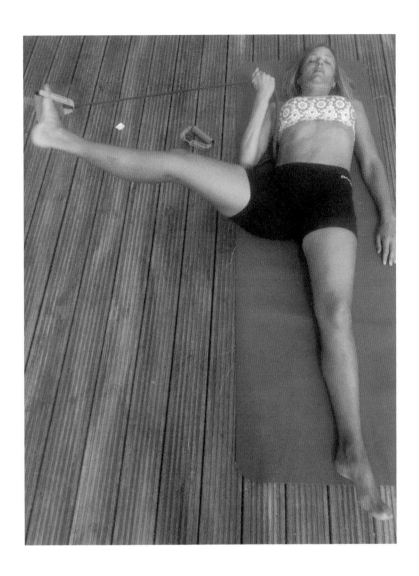

The elevated foot should be held as close to hip height as possible. This will promote a maximum stretch in the groin and inner leg area. Again the head shoulders and neck should remain heavy and relaxed.

CHAPTER 10

Inversions

Feet in the air

Sit with your legs straight out in front of you. Place the resistance band across the top of the foot and then put the handles under the foot and through the inside edges of the feet. Holding the handles in both hands swing your feet into the air keeping your torso and lower back in contact with the ground. Breathe deeply in this pose sinking through your shoulders on the exhalation. When you are ready to come down slowly bring your legs back to the ground.

This is an introduction to the shoulderstand and useful as an alternative for those students who can't practice the shoulderstand, for example, those with neck problems. Any student may simply 'put their feet up' and gain the advantage of inversion to the lower leg without the need to use a wall for assistance.

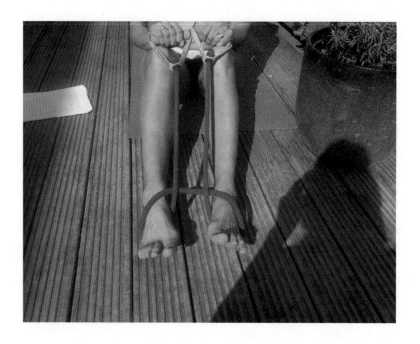

Once again for this posture we use the wrap of the feet method
common to many of the other poses. The band simply goes across the
top of the foot and the handles are then passed through the inside edge
of the feet.

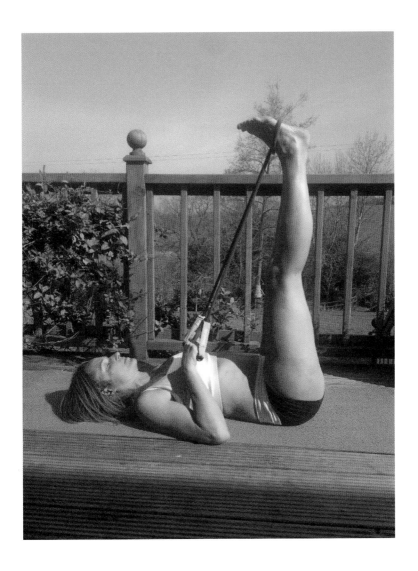

The head and shoulders should remain relaxed and heavy while the legs and feet benefit from the reverse blood flow that this inversion offers. This allows the legs to recuperate and rejuvenate.

Shoulderstand

Sit with your legs straight out in front of you. Place the resistance band across the top of the foot and then put the handles under the foot and through the inside edges of the feet. Holding the handles in both hands bend your knees and swing your feet into the air as if you were attempting a backwards somersault. Keep your upper arms in contact with the ground and hold the handles of the resistance band at chest level. Breathe deeply in this position depressing the upper arms on the exhalation and keeping your chin tucked in and central to the collarbone.

The resistance band is a very valuable piece of equipment to assist with this inversion because the student's feet may push away from the rest of the torso with extra vigour because they may do so against the resistance of the rubber tubing. This enables the legs to remain very straight as well as long and automatically corrects common misalignments found in this popular yoga pose.

The student's shoulders should remain heavy and carry no tension while the neck is tucked in centrally to the collarbone to prevent compression. Monitor how your neck feels in the strong forward bend that this pose offers the cervical vertebrae. Exit the pose if there is any discomfort. This pose relieves stiffness around the shoulders, neck and upper spine. Hips and legs bear no weight and are free from the normal pull of gravity. The pose should feel calming and restful and is perfect for recuperation at the end of a hard day.

When ready to leave this position, let your feet travel in the direction behind of your head to enter the plough pose. Your feet may or may not touch the ground. Let them travel as far as they will. Then straighten your arms on the ground away from your head; this will encourage your neck, shoulder and spine to stretch. Hold this pose for several breaths. Plough pose is a strong stretch for the lower back as it is simply a sitting forward bend performed upside down and hence gravity allows for a deeper forward bend on the lumbar spine. This makes it a very good counterbalance to any compression in the lumber that might have taken place during shoulderstand. It may be beneficial to put the band to one side after plough and put both legs back up into the air and shake the feet vigorously after this sequence. This will free the legs of any residual muscular tension from the bands and loosen them in preparation for relaxation.

In this picture my calves, ankles and feet remain relaxed, and are carried upward by the support from below.

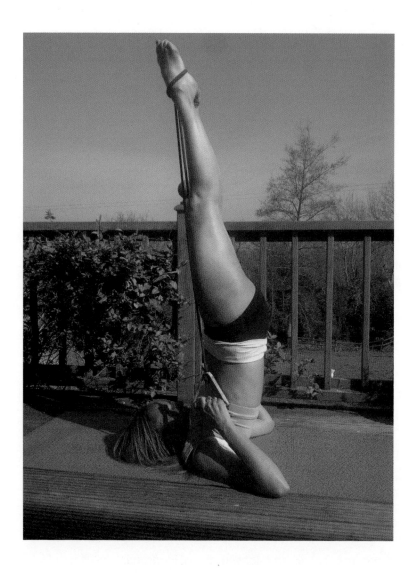

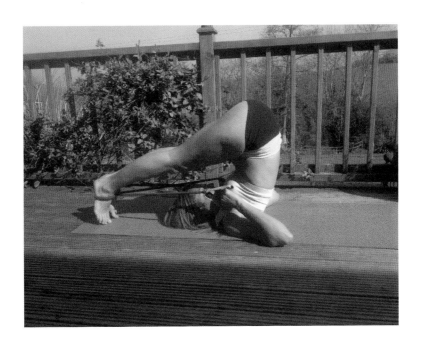

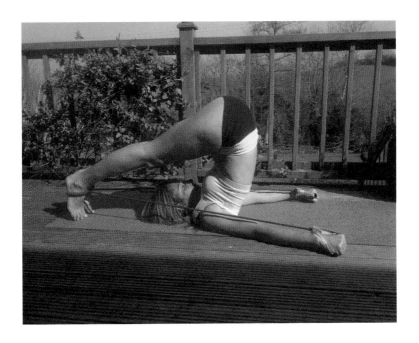

CHAPTER 11

Finishing Class

Deep Relaxation

I ask students to lie on their mats to finish the class and take time to rest and relax their muscles. They should lie on their backs with legs straight and arms at their side's palms up. There should be some space between their limbs and their torso. Eyes should be closed. They should notice how their muscles broaden, soften and lengthen as they relax and sink into their mats. As each student relaxes they will feel heavier and more in contact with the floor. I ask them to acknowledge the experience of being completely supported and encourage them to indulge in the quiet time offered to simply follow the natural rhythm of their breathing. Thoughts may come and go but I try to persuade students to observe them and see them as clouds and let them simply drift by without grasping and engaging with them. This type of concentration takes practice and for some students it may be beneficial to count their breaths or use a mantra. This can be any word that is calming; a Sanskrit one to try is 'SO HAM'. This translates as: I am that.

A student should think 'SO' on the inhalation and 'HAM' on the exhalation. This mudra encourages a student to see through the ego to the quiet still self that is calm, solid and strong. Quiet attention to one's breath clears the mind, and the nervous system shifts from a passive to a relaxation response and a student is able to observe the cumulative effects and benefits from their yoga practice. This is encouraging and stays with them in their transition after the relaxation period back into their busy lives in the great outer world.

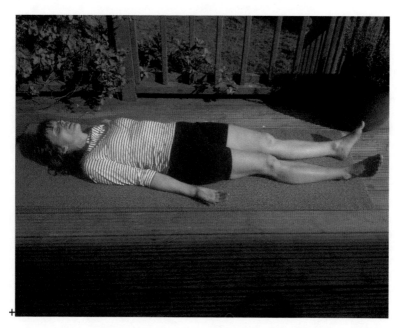

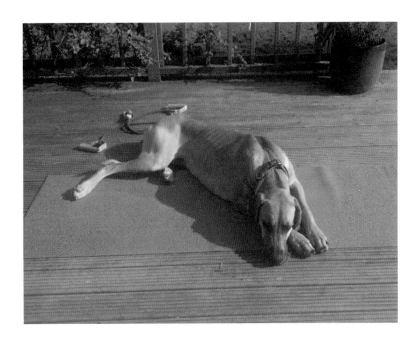

The corpse pose should be done after every yoga practice session and its simplicity is deceptive as it is one of the hardest yoga poses to practice. This is because there is no movement to occupy your thoughts. In lying still and acquainting ourselves with our breath we may glimpse how to meditate and access our true selves. Here we lie alone with simply a mat as our only possession and our breath as our only companion. Allow your breath to be your mind's companion and allow the pull of gravity to let you rest down into your mat. Surrender your body and mind and allow them to be free.

ABOUT THE AUTHOR

Victoria Coven is a Yoga teacher currently living in the Devonshire countryside in the UK. She discovered the benefits that the resistance band could bring to the practice of yoga when using the bands from general fitness and strength training. Using the bands brings a unique benefit to the traditional yoga postures and this book allows students to discover how to incorporate the bands into their daily practice and reap the benefits that they offer to the spine and joints.

Printed in Great Britain
by Amazon.co.uk, Ltd.,
Marston Gate.